I0839867

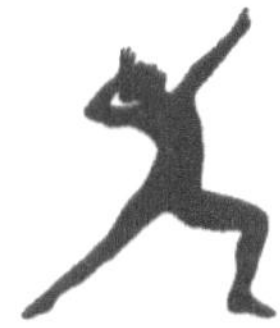

CRAMP AND PAIN FREE

A SIMPLE, PRACTICAL AND SUSTAINABLE SOLUTION

John Dickinson

AUTHOR

Jennifer Mears

EDITOR

ISBN: 9798866375820

GRiTTi Publishing

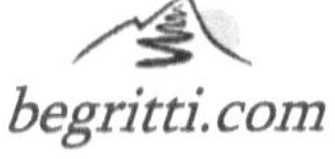

begritti.com

Dedication

This book is dedicated to my friend, Eddie Dykes.

Muscle cramps cost him his life. He tragically never made it back to shore in September 2021, while paddling on Midmar Dam (South Africa).

It could so easily have been me—and, yes, so many others too.

Sadly, my discovery was too late to save Eddie, but for those who continue to suffer, unnecessarily, you could soon be cramp and pain free.

Imagine what's possible?

When your head and heart are done, your spirit still burns brightly deep within. There's always more, but finding this profound inner guidance amidst life's crises—*and heeding it*—is difficult.

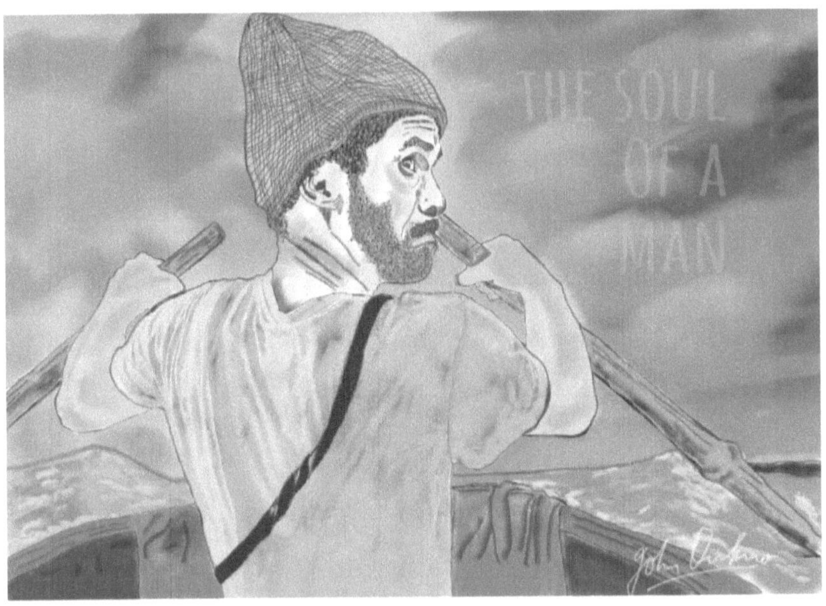

A picture which I painted on my phone while on the CRAMP FREE journey. I was inspired; the inner guidance was irresistible.

CONTENTS

CONTENTS

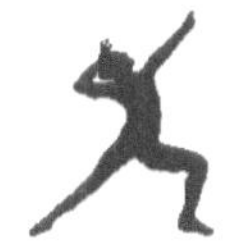

PREFACE

I'm still in awe of what happened that day

Our greatest wish is to live inspired and meaningful lives. Life's greatest challenge is to deliver on this promise to ourselves.

My date with destiny

It's often when we least expect it, that our world-view is turned on its head.

'It's in your genes John. You'll have to live with your cramps.'

But they were wrong.

I chanced upon my cramp-healing solution on 21 October 2021. Within 48 hours I was cramp free, *without the need for any form of ongoing medication.*

I was incredulous. It was scarcely believable; a life-changing discovery.

As a friend put it to me; *'John, you've found the key which everyone's overlooked, and which has given you access to the fathomless depths of a deep-healing vault'.*

More than two years later, at the time of writing, I remain cramp free.

Few would believe that it's true, or even possible. What's truly remarkable is the fact that, at the time, healing my cramps wasn't even on my mind. I was trying to fix my right foot which I'd injured during the initial lockdown period, and then made considerably worse by joining my friends on a hike to the top of South Africa's Drakensberg Mountains, in May 2021.

I'd long since given up on my leg cramps. Their healing was completely fortuitous and incidental. However, now that I more fully understand what happened that day, and given the enormous impact that it's had on my quality of life—*and, yes, my dreams*—it's time to share my discovery.

I trust that you will enjoy your journey into self-healing as much as I have mine. Make no mistake, you will be surprised, and, I hope, inspired…

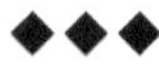

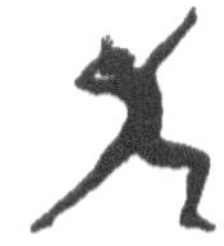

CHAPTER 1

Breaking the shackles of convention

---

*Wellbeing is everything. We have nowhere
else to live, except in our bodies.*

There's nowhere to run

Your body is your permanent mobile home. Wellbeing, or its absence, sits at the very core of how you experience your life.

Although pain and suffering are unavoidable, in most cases there's no need for us to settle for so much of it. If you're up for doing what others won't, then there's every possibility that the CRAMP FREE journey could help you suffer *much* less—and *live* much more.

Becoming cramp and pain free is a real possibility

Have you, like so many millions of others, simply given up and learned to live with the violent pain of foot and leg cramps, and their random occurrence, *especially at night?*

If so, it's important for you to know that what I'm about to share with you, could help you get rid of your cramps—and catalyse a still deeper, self-liberating journey.

The personal cost

Apart from the pain and frustration they cause, leg cramps can rob us of our dreams, negatively impact our relationships, and disturb our sleep patterns.

The significance of my discovery

I'd tried every trick in the conventional and alternative healing book, but nothing had worked. I was getting little sleep and risking serious health consequences.

When I chanced upon my cramp-healing solution—while trying to heal my foot, which I'd hurt during the initial Lockdown period—I immediately understood its significance.

It was as if I'd been plagued by cramps for so many years—*and then hurt my foot*—so that I could help other sufferers around the globe connect with what they'd always hoped they would find, but never had.

The choice

Who you've become is the consequence of the choices you've made.

Who you become will be determined by the choices you make.

You're always just one *active* decision away from a different future.

The truly miraculous part of the cramp-healing process is this; that once you've made that choice, and healed your cramps, it's impossible not to find yourself on a life-shifting journey like no other. The mechanism is such that it spontaneously catalyses within us, what I'm now calling *'the deep-healing response'.* It's a cascade of restorative responses; physical, emotional and spiritual.

Once your wellbeing, which you thought was in a permanent downward spiral, is on a sustained upward trajectory, your outlook will shift. That's when you'll step out of the grind and back into the flow of possibility.

I can't know for how long, or how much, you've suffered, but I'm sure it's long enough to know that it's not how you want to spend the rest of your life.

The sign

At the time of my cramp-healing discovery, on 21 October 2021, I was helping my friend, Ross McLean, run his boutique guesthouse in Paternoster, on South Africa's West Coast.

Still high on the euphoria of finding myself miraculously cramp and pain free, I did 'the breakfast run'—as always. It was while chatting to one of the couples in the restaurant that, unexpectedly, they turned the tables and began asking me about my life.

Unable to contain myself, I shared the story of my cramp-healing discovery. I recall being astonished to discover that they were both doctors (another coincidence?); Dr Paree Amod, a GP, and Dr Willie Koen, a cardiothoracic surgeon who specialised in heart transplants and new heart treatment technologies.

They were as fascinated by my cramp healing solution, as I was by their experiences as medical doctors. To their great credit they did not simply dismiss the findings of a layman, but instead suggested that *'it was logical and made perfect sense'.*

This was all the encouragement I needed to share my discovery with the world.

◆◆◆

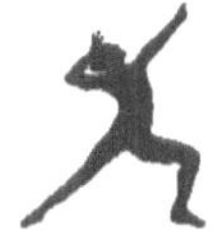

CHAPTER 2

Journey into possibility

The day we are born, our lives begin. The day we understand why, our lives are transformed.

Early October 2021

Even before my breakthrough healing experience, running Ross's boutique guesthouse had turned into an unbelievably uplifting time in my life—despite my foot pain, and the cramps I was experiencing.

I've often wondered whether, by taking a leap of fear and faith, and stepping into the flow of that guesthouse (I'd never been in hospitality before), I inadvertently raised myself up for the series of miracles which were to follow.

I'd awaken each morning, shattered, after yet another night of leaping out of bed with mind-bending foot, calf and hamstring cramps, and wishing that I could sleep for another five hours. I'd then force myself through a repetitive, hard, mind-clearing, life-coping, yoga routine. In fact, it was hardly yoga; I took to calling it *'Johga'* (John's yoga). Despite the unresolved pain in my foot, I naively pushed on, somehow convincing myself—as I had since the initial Lockdown period—that it would sort itself out.

I can recall looking at myself in the mirror and being surprised by how frail and gaunt I looked. My legs were way too thin. A friend had taken to calling me 'stick man', and that had been four months prior, shortly after I'd returned from the top-of-the-Drakensberg hike, which had proved to be the last straw. I'm sure, had she seen me in my more recent incarnation, that she'd have found an even more apt name for me, like *the invisible man*'!

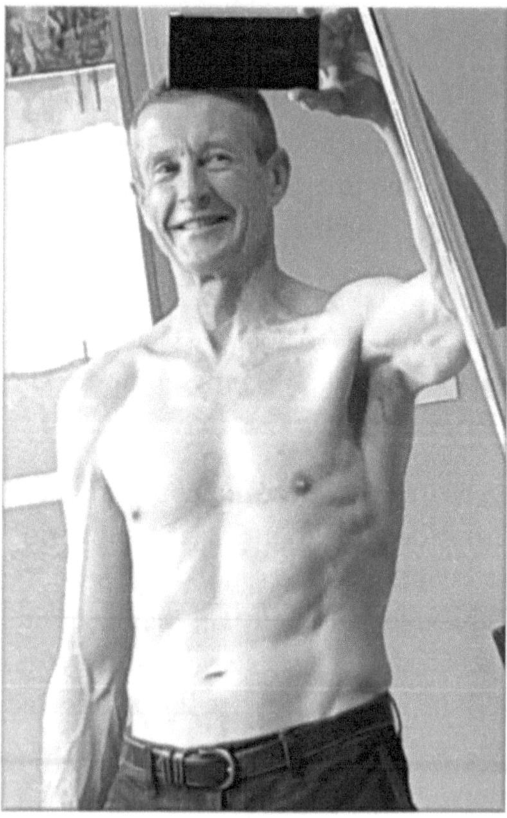

I took this photo during the initial Lockdown period, because a friend had asked what yoga was doing for me. Looking at it now, I can see where 'stick man' came from!

As much as I knew that I needed to move to stay healthy, I also needed to move carefully, and not too much, if I was to avoid the worst of the cramps that night. My life was narrowing. My dreams were becoming fogged and clogged.

From being about the most active and positive person I'd ever known, my life had become increasingly confined and small. I couldn't escape the fact that I was in little more than survival mode.

And yet, somehow, I recall stepping into each day, excited about what might unfold. Little did I know that, apart from the incredible people I'd meet, the ultimate miracle would turn out to be the unexpected healing of my leg cramps.

Supposedly, we're stuck with cramps as we age

The more I'd read over the years, the more I'd resigned myself to believing that leg cramps were one of the inevitable costs of aging. It seemed that most people, at some stage, suffered from them, *especially at night.* For many, their story was like mine; the anticipation of another agonizing night ahead, with no end in sight.

I couldn't even drive too far, knowing that using the clutch and accelerator would stress my muscles and trigger the most severe cramps that night, if not before.

I was at a loss. It dawned on me that, at some level, my cramps had even cost me my marriages. Can you imagine being married to somebody who jumped out of bed like a jack-in-the-box, five to twenty times a night, every night?

Your deep-healing rite of passage

In one way or another, we're all stuck with who we've been convinced into believing we are, what I call our *'synthetic identity'.* Fortunately, it's circumstantial—*not genetic*—and so, with high levels of motivation and self-accountability, we can choose to shift it.

As you kick off your own self-healing journey, you'll find yourself listening intently to what your life and your body say to you about where you're at. Your circumstances will directly speak to you.

The cramp-healing process will provide you with a unique vehicle for a very personal, self-generated, enquiry into your life. In your own time and at your own pace, you can breathe, take stock and act with conscious deliberation.

You'll find that it's the unexpectedness of the healing, together with the inevitable journey into self-enquiry and possibility, which has the potential to catapult you into still higher levels of healing and meaning. It's like a rite of passage into a more purposeful future. The healing process awakens within us a deep desire to embrace new possibilities and a higher level of *being* in this world.

As poet William Ernest Henley so aptly said, *'I am the master of my fate; I am the captain of my soul.*

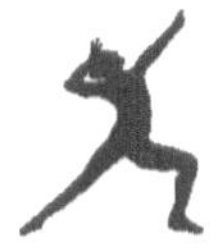

CHAPTER 3

The origin of my cramps?

All men die. Few men ever really live.

From the movie, 'Braveheart'

Looking back

I've always been an avid adventurer and sports enthusiast.

Over the course of my 62 years, I've put my body through countless leg, foot, back and neck damaging incidents.

Struggles at school

Junior school included my infamous attempt to do a somersault on a cement floor at the age of twelve. Having never attempted such an acrobatic manoeuvre in my life before, our impromptu house-play in front of the whole Merchiston boarding establishment, proved too tempting.

Unknowingly, I managed to break off bony processes from my lumbar spine, causing instability in my lower back. This was only diagnosed—as an old injury—ten years later, when my back was X-rayed for the first time, following a rugby concussion at university. I had what's called a spondylolisthesis, with its characteristic 'scotty-dog fractures'.

At the time, I recall being sent to bed by the matron, embarrassed and in agony, with a headache pill. I then lived with the intermittent, sometimes extreme pain, of pinched nerves. Yes, I tried to explain what was wrong to the medical fraternity at the time, but nobody bothered to investigate further, and physiotherapy was in its infancy back then.

Sometimes, I struggled to bend down and make my bed, without my back going into spasm.

Only now have I made the (possible) connection between this injury so early in my life, and the cramps that I went on to live with for so many years.

When it came to running races at school, I seldom won, but I took myself to the brink of complete exhaustion every time. On one occasion, I can remember pulling chunks of turf out of the Maritzburg College athletics field. This was the consequence of suffering with severe cramps, after having given it my all in the 800 and 1500-metre races, which were run in quick succession.

Into the unknown

Having done my best to impress my peers at school, I waved good-bye to friends and family and began my compulsory two years of military service.

Contextually, 1979 wasn't a good time to be in the army. The apartheid years were at their peak and the war effort on South Africa's borders and beyond was in full stride. Driven by ego and the promise of adventure, I chose to try out for an elite paratrooping unit with a high barrier to entry. And, no, I never divulged that I was still at risk of suffering from occasional (sometimes extreme) lower back pain. It would have meant an instant dismissal from the selection process, and a loss of face in front of my peers.

I'd been told that only the strongest survived. Having begun the journey, I was prepared only to succeed, or die trying.

Those who failed the various stages of the selection process were given what we called an RTU ('Return To Unit'). You wore it, if only in your mind, as a badge of shame, for the rest of your life. This was never an option for me. It would have been too great a cross to bear. As it turned out, our level of core fitness was so high, that it probably saved me from the lower back pain which would otherwise have seen me X-rayed and RTUed!

No end to my ego

The Rag Relay was an annual event at the university I attended. It involved relay teams racing each other on the Comrades Marathon route between Pietermaritzburg and Durban, in South Africa.

Selected for one of the teams, I found myself in the very unfortunate position of being fifty metres behind Speedy, at my takeover point. Speedy, running for one of the opposition teams, had been my wife-to-be's previous boyfriend. The thought of him beating me was unthinkable, even if he did have a good head-start.

We had to race each other in very hot conditions, for 7km, up an undulating hill to the next changeover. I eventually caught Speedy, stayed on his heels for a while, and then burst past in a decisive move designed to silence him. I waved nonchalantly as I cantered past, and then appeared to accelerate effortlessly away.

It probably never mattered in the slightest to Speedy, but for me it was a question of life and death. He was not to know it, but I'd just given it my all. Once safely past, and having glanced back to make sure that he had no answers, I slowed and ran the final stretch on empty—losing most of my vision over the final 20 metres, and cramping badly on the drive home.

Still keen to impress, I jumped onto my steel, 1970's style Raleigh bicycle, at 3:00 am one morning, and attempted to ride from Pietermaritzburg to her family's farm in Swartberg, KwaZulu-Natal. For those familiar with the route, you'll know just how mountainous it is, and how hot the Umkomaas Valley becomes, mid-summer. Had I made it, it would have been close to a 200km ride. Before that morning, I'd never cycled more than 15km at any one time.

With four slices of bread and butter taken from the university cafeteria the night before, and a large bottle of water, I set off with a small rucksack. I made it just past Underberg (130km), before having to turn back, admit defeat, and phone her father from the local hotel. The cramps hit as, shattered, I climbed into his monstrous Ford Fairlane for the trip to the farm.

From there, I upped the impressing stakes still further, by competing in ultra-marathons, in particular the 89 km

Comrades Marathon, in 1984. But I was plagued by cramps near the ends of these races, and long into the night. Driving home was always a stop-start affair—slamming on brakes, leaping out and trying to prevent the cramps from biting too deeply.

Paragliding pioneers

Once I'd left university, married the amazing young woman I'd put in so much effort to impress, and having had enough of being a corporate misfit, I moved on to help pioneer paragliding in South Africa.

My best was teaching people to fly. I'll always recall the anxiety on their faces before their first proper flight, followed by the utter disbelief—and joy—when they'd successfully pulled it off.

On one occasion, my friend Michael and I spent the day running up and down a mountain, teaching students to fly. That afternoon I dived into a swimming pool and cramped instantly, from my torso down. Michael had to rescue me. But nobody could help me as I lay on the side of the pool, writhing and groaning in agony.

Later that evening, alone, after the others headed off to dinner, I was forced to endure a second round of extreme cramps. They eventually become unbearable. I had to crawl to the phone and call a doctor. He injected me with a muscle relaxant which finally did the trick, but, as always, it was temporary.

The ultimate price

And then, sometime in July 1990, I managed to step off a cliff with a foreign paraglider which I'd been persuaded to test fly, and it all went horribly wrong. As usual, I'd not spared a thought for my own safety, but instead had been hell-bent on pleasing and impressing. This time, though, it very nearly cost me my life.

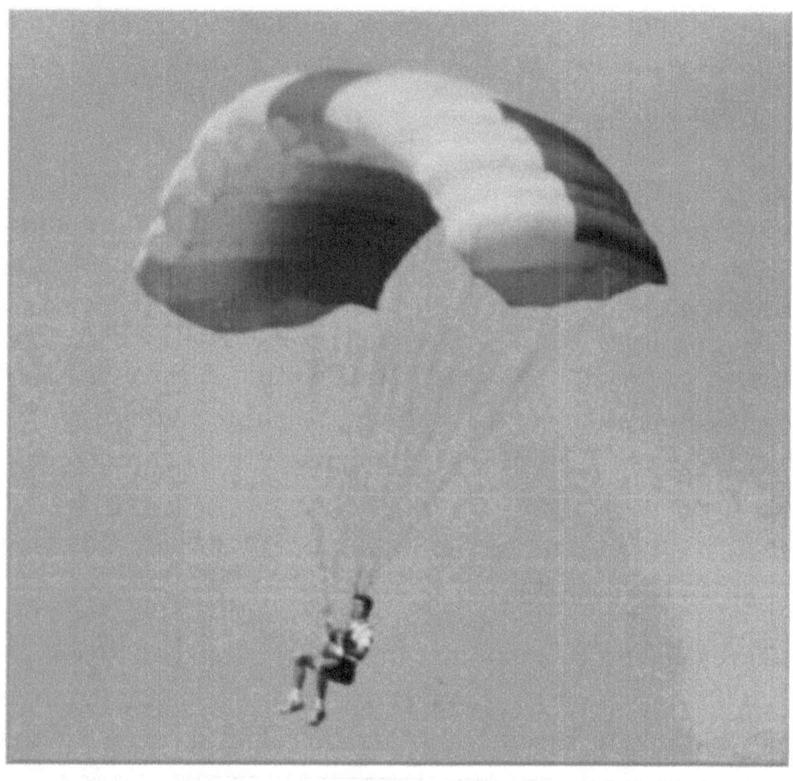

Neither helmets nor reserve chutes back then. That's me, free as a bird—at least for a while...

I over-cooked a turn and collapsed the canopy. I fell hard, knocking myself unconscious in the process.

There's no doubt that my paratrooping experience saved my life that day. It had taught me to force myself into the right shape for the crash-landing (elbows in, chin on chest, feet together and watch the ground). Only, this time, I went one better; I closed my eyes just before the impact, and went limp.

It wasn't anything I'd ever planned to do. I just did it, instinctively. It made all the difference. Had I remained rigid and upright, my hips would have popped, and my spine would have crumpled.

As it was, I landed like a limp rag-doll, and pulled off an impossible medical procedure in the process. The accident literally smashed my 'dislocated spine' (from my early childhood somersault), back into place. This was confirmed by an X-ray, which I wish I'd kept.

I was then advised that if I could keep things stable until I was in my 40s, the floating remains of the spinal processes (the so-called 'scotty dog' fractures), would slowly re-attach themselves to my spine. I have no idea whether this actually happened, but I can happily say that I've lived with relatively little back pain since the accident, which could so easily have ended my life.

It took many years to fully recover. The orthopaedic surgeon who examined me at the time, advised that I'd probably walk with a limp for the rest of my life, and that running was out of the question. Fortunately, none of this came to pass. I went on to walk limp-free, and I'm still running to this day—*now pain and cramp free!*

Mountains calling

Having 'crashed and burned', and on the long road back to recovery, Michael and I took up adventure biking. There were many minor crashes, as we resurrected old bikes and explored further and further afield, but the biggest and most painful—with enduring consequences—happened in a remote area of the Lesotho Highlands.

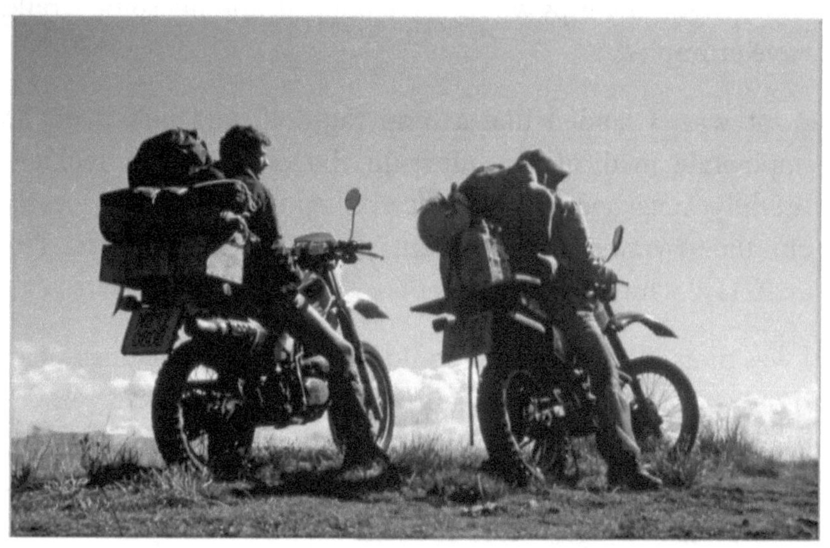

Somewhere in Lesotho. At the time it was our favourite adventure playground.

We still had a difficult pass to descend. Failing to register that the approaching puddle was in fact half a metre deep, with a vertical wall on the far side, I hit it at more than 60km/hour.

The front wheel stopped dead and I was promptly launched into an unplanned flight over the handlebars. My left foot hooked in the crash-bar, twisting itself, breaking bones and badly damaging my calf. The foot healed, but it became increasingly distorted as the years passed.

Michael sent me the picture below, suggesting that my foot was sore today, because of this accident that took place more than 30 years ago. However, if you study the image, you can see that it's in fact my left foot which is damaged, while my most recent injury—during lockdown—was to my right foot.

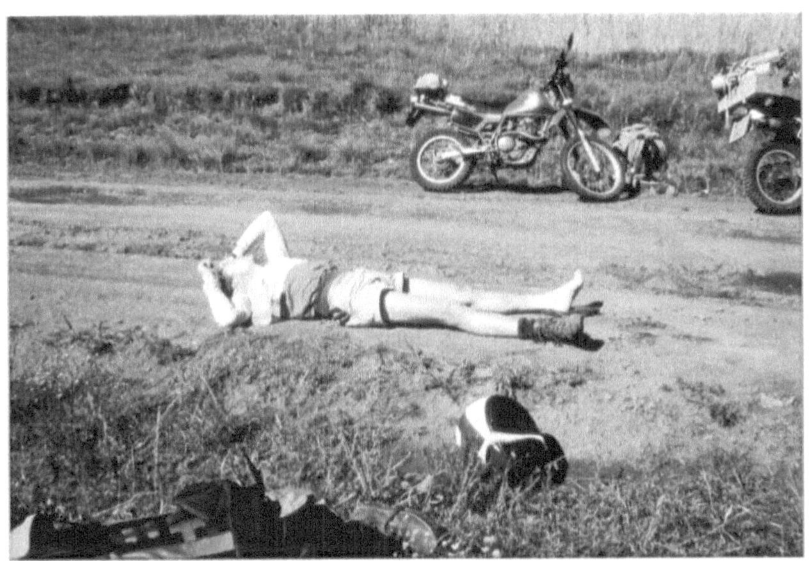

The aftermath of a good crash! In fact, I was very fortunate that it wasn't much worse.

Of course, it's very possible that in compensating for my damaged left foot over the years, I had inadvertently damaged my right one.

On the brink of despair

The final cramping straw was that now infamous hike to the top of the Drakensberg Mountains in South Africa. I couldn't resist the lure of yet another adventure, with my friends Rupert, Mike and Thomas.

I'd known before we left Johannesburg at five that morning, that it'd be risky. My foot hurt, a lot, and I hadn't done enough preparation. But nothing could have prepared me for that first night.

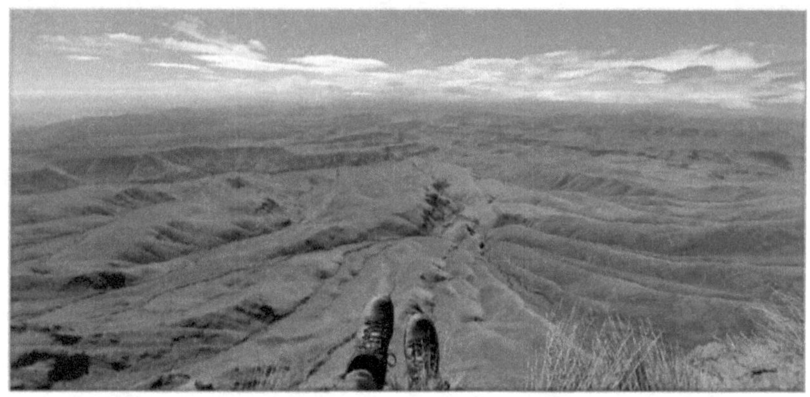

It was worth the effort, despite the challenges.
Our view from the top of the Drakensberg.

Jumping up for the umpteenth time and hitting my head on the roof of the cave, I found myself reflecting on just how diabolical my circumstances had become. I was 60 years old, lying in a sleeping bag at the mouth of a cave at nearly 3000 metres—in freezing cold temperatures, and in the face of a howling gale—and being assaulted by violent foot, calf and hamstring cramps every few minutes.

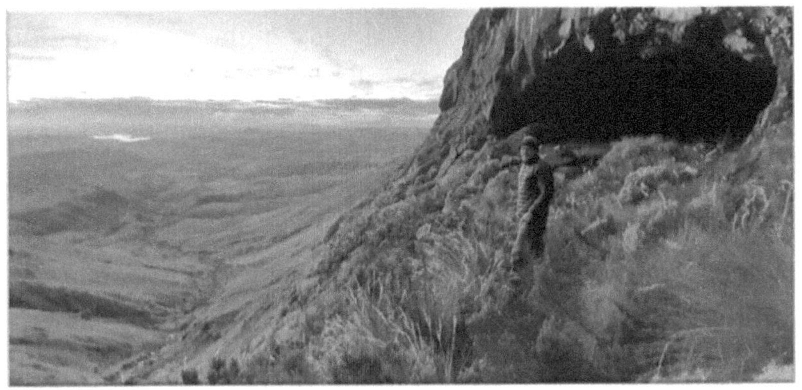

Thomas standing in front of the infamous cave, the morning after.

I had no choice but to leap out of my sleeping bag with great speed, hitting my head on the roof of the cave every time, so quick did my exit need to be. If I didn't catch them within seconds, the cramps would bite so deeply that I couldn't help screaming into the wind. My calves and hamstrings would bunch up into metal balls and my foot would contort itself into an impossible ballet pose. First my right leg, and then the left, alternately. Fortunately, never both at the same time!

With each of my exits, I'd curse and groan, and my sleeping bag would be blown against the far wall. My friends would turn away, dig deeper into their sleeping bags, and pull their pillows over their heads. There was nothing they could do to help. I recall thinking, in those moments, that it would be my last big hike.

Staring down the barrel

And that had been the story of my life for nearly 40 years. I'd often leap out of bed five to ten times a night, and even more frequently when I'd been exercising hard, or recovering from an accident.

And yet, somehow, throughout those years, I'd always seen cramping as a temporary problem. That was until early October 2021, when it'd become pretty much untenable.

I could no longer kid myself into believing that my cramps were temporary. I had to accept that something was terribly wrong, and that nobody—neither in the medical profession, nor outside of it—had an answer.

I'd tried every trick in the conventional and alternative healing book. None had worked. NONE. Not magnesium, not B vitamins, not potassium (bananas), not table salt, not calcium, not tissue salts, not hydration, not physiotherapy, not chiropractic therapy, not acupuncture. NOTHING. And my life, as it stood right then, was being seriously compromised.

I was getting little sleep and risking serious health consequences. One's brain and heart don't take kindly to not having the chance to fully recharge themselves every 24 hours. For that matter, neither does any organ in your body. They're all adversely affected.

My life, quite literally, was at risk. And it could only get worse. It would be a slow spiral into oblivion, with no about-turn option. My health was, for the first time, out of my control. *Completely.*

I was scared, to put it mildly. Despite priding myself on always finding a way through—and being an inspiring role model to others—this time round I had no answers.

28

Soft soles and high heels are like fast food for your feet.

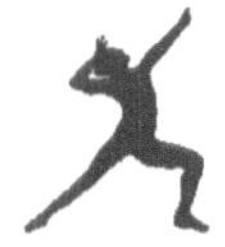

CHAPTER 4

Deep insight—*ignored!*

To find your mission in life is to discover the intersection between your heart's deep gladness, and the world's deep hunger.

Frederick Beekner

Anticipation

Sitting there in the Alternative Healing Therapist's Rooms, *twenty years ago,* with all the electrodes glued to my head and body, I was expectant but doubtful. I could neither see how the process could reveal anything to the therapist sitting behind her computer, nor how it could benefit my aches and pains. The technology was new to me. I was only there because a well-meaning friend had persuaded me that it would be a worthwhile experience.

Back then I was busy. I was running mountains, paddling rivers, exploring oceans, and riding endless trails on mountain and motor bikes. I would fall, wrench muscles, or crash, often.

I was sore and, yes, cramping, constantly. At times, the only way I could describe the pain to my friends (family didn't listen!) was, *'It's like my bones are cramping'.*

I was there because of the general all-over pain that I lived with, rather than my muscle cramps in particular. They'd long been a given in my life, even though, bizarrely, I'd never seen them as permanent.

I'll never forget the therapist in conversation with me while tapping away on her keyboard, and then, suddenly, silence. I looked up to see that her face had become ashen, and there were beads of perspiration on her forehead.

Instantly on high alert, I wondered what she could possibly have seen on her screen. As the seconds dragged on, I became increasingly alarmed.

About to jump up and see for myself, I realised that it wouldn't be a clever move. The electrodes were pouring from me. I couldn't get up without disturbing them.

Finally, after what seemed like an age, she asked, very quietly and tentatively, *'Have you had an accident?'*

I couldn't think of anything recent, so feeling puzzled, I said, *'No'*, and then as an afterthought, *'What sort of accident?'*

She replied immediately, *'A big one!'*

'Yes!', I replied, instantly. 'I had a paragliding accident ten years ago. It nearly cost me my life.'

But how could she be *'seeing'* an accident that I'd had ten years before? I was amazed, but still very concerned about what she'd found.

Visibly relieved at my reply, it was only later that she revealed why she'd been so alarmed. Her screen, as she then showed me, had blinking red exclamation marks all over it, signifying either a fatal diagnosis, or the consequence of a major historical accident. In my case, it was almost certainly the latter.

On the back of the information that she gleaned from the electrodes, she was able to play back the story of my life, and provide me with useful rehabilitation guidelines. Of course, as is so often the case with these things, I thanked her profusely, but ignored her sage advice. Her wisdom was wasted on me, until now.

Our bodies record the story of our lives

Our bodies are like history books. We write, scribble, dance, love, play, paint, or force—whether by choice or circumstance—a new chapter into our bodies, every day of our lives. Our activities, thoughts and feelings, are dutifully recorded in every living cell in our bodies. The outward stories—the ones we live—together with their associated memories and emotions, become hard-wired into our cellular history books.

Now, *in the current context,* I get it, that this remarkable process had revealed the partial breakdown of my body's matrix of connective tissue—*or fascia*—and, with it, the loss of some of its innate intelligence.

My body, as is the case with everybody else's, had, over time, been battered by a unique mix of physical and emotional traumas, and marinated in a lifetime of stress, anxiety and dietary abuse. My muscle cramps, with their associated pains and consequences, were but one more unfortunate spin-off of the story of my life so far.

An unused gift (I still shake my head in disbelief)

I've achieved all of my healing using the technology and deep-healing techniques that were gifted to me by a long-standing friend, Vanessa, long before my date with the therapist. But, as with the therapist's advice, I'd failed to use her gift—until now, that is—despite knowing that it would help me deal with my persistent physical pains and recurring injuries (I'd had no idea that it would help me heal my cramps). I guess it's in our nature to spend our lives preparing to live, one day. I'd always known that I'd eventually get there, but I never had.

The answer to my cramps had been staring me in the face for all those years. All I had to do was open my eyes and make the connection that, bizarrely, nobody else had either.

Professional athletes use similar tools and technology to help maintain their optimal performance. They're also being used by therapists to help people relieve pain and stiffness, but until now their specific application as a cramp-healing solution has not been documented (as far as I have been able to establish).

At first, I was at a loss as to why, given how effective it has proved to be. However, now that I've been cramp-free for more than two years, the reason, as I see it, is all too evident.

It's such a simple and apparently innocent solution

The foam roller is a simple and very effective cramp-healing solution. However, it requires a more thorough, consistent, *and intense,* self-healing application of the same techniques used by athletes and therapists.

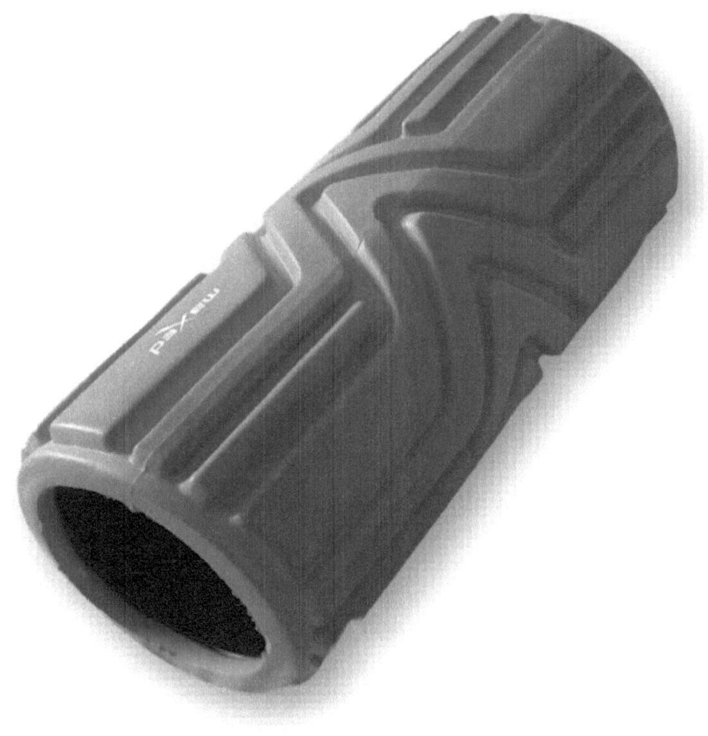

The foam-roller. An incredibly effective self-healing tool.

It is the initial, intense, 'breakthrough' application of the technology—*aimed specifically at cramps*—which is the game-changer. I was very fortunate to, quite incidentally, hit a sufficiently high level of intensity, that it sparked the healing of both my foot, and my leg cramps. At the time my foot was so sore that, in my desperation, I'd been fully prepared to put in the painful, self-healing effort required.

That's not to say, though, that the intense, breakthrough experience, can't be spread out using a more gentle approach, over a much longer time period. I'll talk more about this shortly.

What exactly is a foam roller?

In case you're not familiar with a foam roller, it's either made from solid but compressible foam, of various diameters (the average is about 14cm), or the foam is wrapped around a thick, plastic, pipe-like core.

In my experience, the *solid* foam rollers are a little more forgiving—i.e., less painful—and so they're a good place to start. The 'hard core' rollers are just that, *harder.* Some of them are even ribbed, or knobbly, providing for a much deeper, more intense, and effective, self-massage experience.

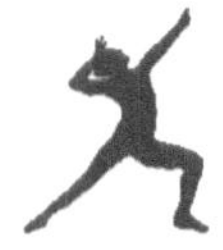

CHAPTER 5

The healing

It's your life. Go get it...

Preparation

I healed the cumulative effects of 50 plus years of self-inflicted physical and emotional abuse (most of it was fun at the time) and, incidentally, my leg cramps—in the space of just 48 hours. To achieve this, I had to push my self-defeating voice aside, dig deep, and endure a fair amount of physical pain. The consequences, aside from my cramp-free life, have been nothing short of astonishing.

However, to benefit from my technique's extraordinary capacity for deep healing, you too will need to ignore your self-limiting voice, and prepare your mind for what's to come. The good news is that you can choose how much pain and discomfort you're prepared to endure at any one time.

I chose to heal myself in just 48 hours, but you can do it over a week or two, if you choose. It depends on how you're feeling, your fitness levels, and how quickly you'd like to free yourself from your pain and suffering.

Whatever your choice, I encourage you to push through and keep moving. Ultimately, momentum—*not speed*—is what counts.

It's not a race. It's a life-transforming opportunity which must take place at your own pace and in your own time, once you're equipped with a foam-roller and the necessary insights and techniques.

The mysterious wonder of our fascia

We've known about the existence of *fascia* for thousands of years, but it's only since 2017—with advances in imaging and research techniques—that it has gradually emerged as probably the most important, the biggest, *and the most ignored* organ in our bodies.

My own experience of working with fascia has convinced me that it's the key to cramps, deep healing, mobility, *and wellbeing.*

Our fascia is a three-dimensional, *nerve-infused* network of uninterrupted, multi-layered, connective tissue. It connects every part of our body with every other part, including our skin, organs, nerves, muscles, tendons and bones.

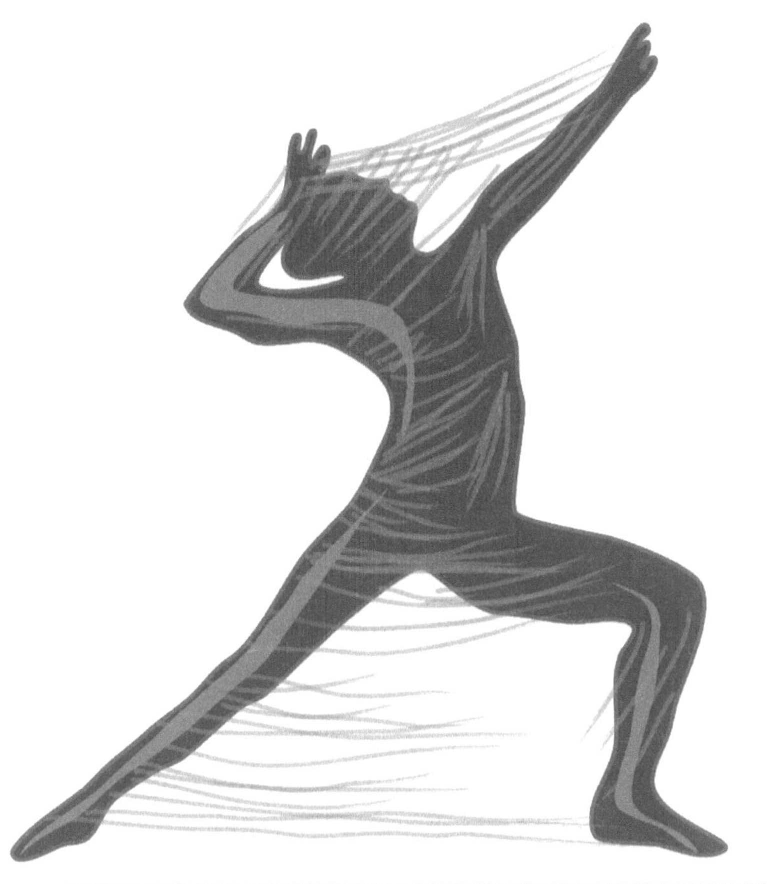

My artistic interpretation of our fascia. It's impossible to adequately convey the magic of this matrix of 'intelligent' connective tissue, which both holds us together and helps orchestrate our every movement.

In concert with our musculoskeletal system, our fascia provides for our exceptional strength, flexibility and mobility.

However, the combination of ageing, sitting, stress, anxiety, depression, abuse, muscle overuse, bad diets, and trauma, all take their toll. Our fascia's physical properties—*smooth, slippery, strong, intelligent, and flexible*—are gradually compromised. It dries up and loses many of its innate capabilities. It becomes like a hardened chamois leather, with which we wash our cars—once it's been left in the sun to dry.

The consequence is that we become increasingly inflexible, lose co-ordination, say goodbye to our mobility, become ever more anxious and narrow in our outlook—*and we get cramps.* Our wellbeing is compromised.

Rebooting

We need to find a way to restore and rehydrate our fascia, melt the scars and adhesions in our muscles and tendons, renew our nerve-ends, and re-establish a rich blood flow to these elements. We need a system reboot of sorts, to ensure that everything gets back to working as synchronously as it used to.

It's much like a magnet which loses its magnetic capacity, until its microscopic elements are forcibly pulled back into alignment by a much more powerful magnet. We need to find the equivalent of that 'much more powerful magnet', which will help us restore our original functionality.

Incredibly, such a solution is available, using the foam roller as our rebooting tool of choice.

The breakthrough and its origins in my injured right foot

On 21 October 2021, I found myself in the small makeshift gym in the guesthouse, going through my normal workout routine. My workouts were gradually decreasing in intensity because of my foot pain and the disturbing knowledge that any over-reaching would lead to even more severe leg cramps that night.

At the time, I wasn't focused on fixing my leg cramps. I had accepted them as permanent. I was really looking to heal my very painful right foot, which I've already alluded to on several occasions.

Two years back, I stayed with some close friends during the initial COVID-19 Lockdown. I committed to taking my friend, Pierre, through a daily yoga/workout routine.

It was quite a hectic process. Working with Pierre every day, motivated me to up the ante! With some of the exercises—skipping and plyometrics, in particular (crouching and then jumping onto a deck, and back down)—my foot became noticeably much more painful.

I simply ignored it. We were having too much fun and making great headway. And then, stupidly, I took part in the hike which I referred to earlier in the book.

Looking back, it was obvious that my right foot had been stewing in a lifetime of cumulative traumas: kick-starting large-bore, four-stroke motorbikes, kicking balls, twisting, sprinting, wrenching, jumping, falling—and so much more.

Conventional wisdom suggested rest and foot spas, and, yes, you've guessed, lotions and potions, massage and acupuncture. In extreme cases, it was even suggested that I should immobilize my foot in a cast or plastic boot. This simply wasn't an option for me. I needed to be fully mobile, even if I was gradually losing what little mobility I had left.

I recall sitting on the mat and using my thumb to knead around my foot, and up into the tendons above my ankle. Everything was inflamed and sore.

The tendons which wound their way around the outside of my ankle were much bigger than the ones in my left foot. My whole foot was extremely painful to the touch.

The incidental moment that changed my life

As I sat there contemplating what to do, I spied an orange foam roller lying in the corner of the room. Most of us are familiar with foam rollers, but few of us have ever used one—*properly*. We either don't know how to use them, or we've discovered that they're too painful to be taken seriously!

Using a foam roller

The idea is to position your body in such a way that you can use the foam roller to *'roll out'* all the kinks, knots, adhesions, scars, pains—*and cramps*—in your feet, legs, glutes, hips, back (carefully), neck (carefully), face, jaw, head, arms and shoulders. *Everywhere!*

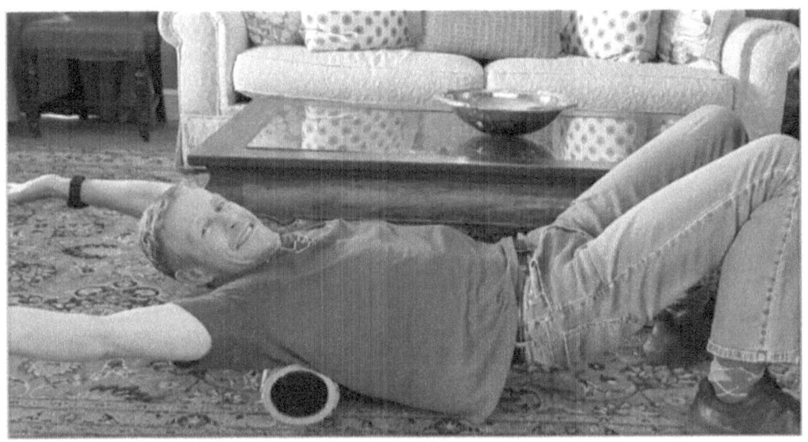

It's supposed to be a good maintenance routine for all of us. For athletes, it helps them avoid injuries and maintain optimal performance. If you're a cramp sufferer, it's the solution you've been waiting for.

You can use a single foam roller for everything, but there are now many variations with more specific applications—for your feet, face and head, for example.

I'm not aware of many people who've voluntarily used their foam rollers. The tiny percentage of those who do use them, do so mostly under supervision and duress, during a Pilates class or equivalent—while mouthing silent curses! Very few of us use them to their full potential, because of how much they hurt.

But it doesn't have to hurt!

Once you've worked out how to modulate the pressure, you'll be able to use it without the pain we're so scared of. That's when you'll begin to experience the foam roller's amazing capacity for catalysing the deep-healing response. Use it consistently, and you'll access ever deeper levels of healing.

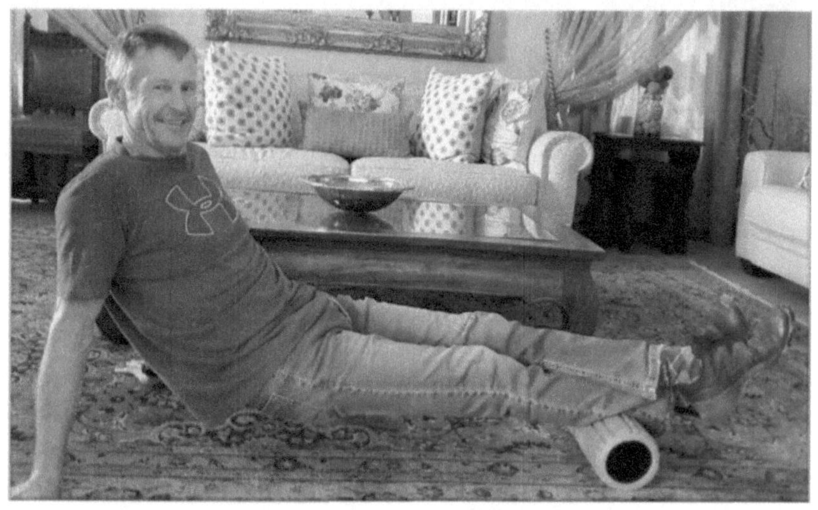

It doesn't make sense, that something which hurts so much can heal so miraculously.

Clearly, very few have managed to break through into that next dimension, where the deep-healing response kicks in. We buy foam rollers because they're trendy to have, but 99% of them lie around idle and unused.

Amazing things start happening

Without much thought, I picked up the roller and positioned it next to my right leg. Then I lay on my right side, placed my right elbow on the mat, leveraged myself into a side-plank (left leg on top of my right)—and pulled the foam roller under the lower part of my right leg. I then gently lowered myself onto the roller and let my feet leave the floor.

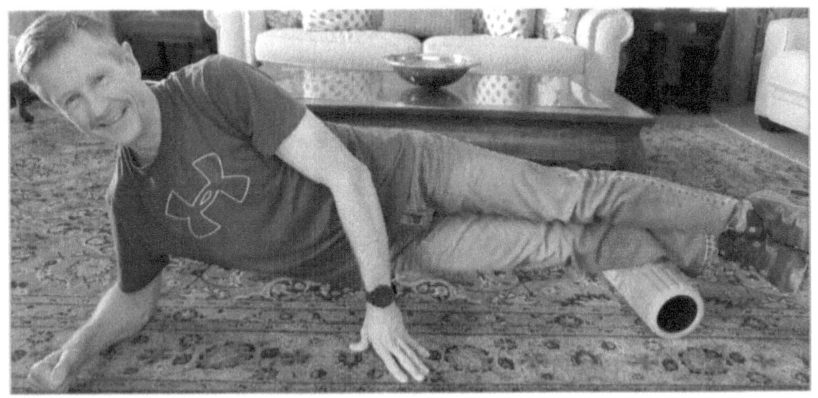

*I then gently lowered myself onto the roller
and let my feet leave the floor.*

Momentarily, my full weight was on my elbow at one end of the mat, and on my inflamed tendons at the other. The pain was unbelievable.

I quickly placed my left foot back on the floor and raised my right leg above the roller. In a flash I knew that I'd found the solution to my foot problem. The whole picture of what was going on inside my sore foot, and why it wasn't healing, became perfectly clear. In that moment of insight, it dawned on me that my foot would never heal, as long as my lower leg's fascia, tendons and calf muscles were inflamed and compromised, with restricted blood flow and possibly even damaged nerve-ends. These mission-critical elements simply could not do what they were supposed to, while they were in this sub-optimal condition.

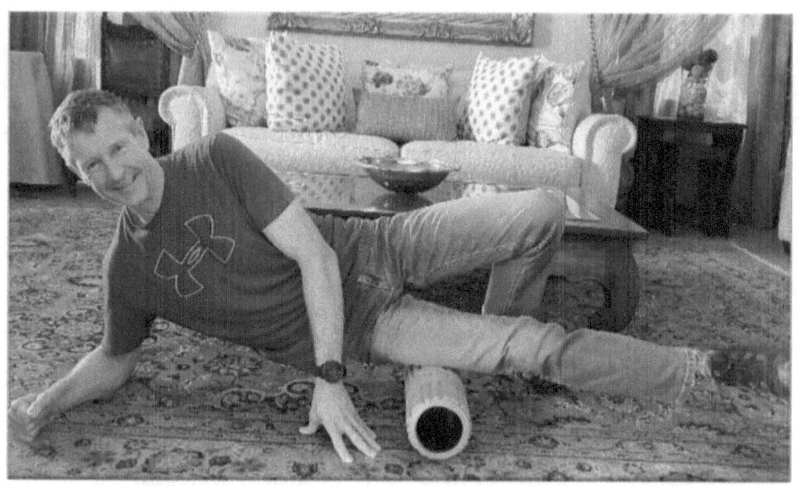

My foot tendons and fascia—already damaged through overuse—had to consistently 'stretch' beyond their design limits, to compensate for the elements in my lower leg not being capable of doing what they were supposed to. In short, it became obvious to me that the problem lay within the fascia, muscles and tendons in my lower leg, and not in the foot itself. Finally, I had closed the causal loop.

The healing work begins

I immediately went to work with the foam roller—the one with the hard inner core (I didn't know the difference back then)—on my right leg. The pain was indescribable, and I could only stay up on my elbow for short stints at a time. I was quickly exhausted by the pain and strain, but excited beyond words. I knew that I was onto something.

Interestingly, while I was focusing on healing my painful right foot, I still hadn't made the connection with my leg cramps.

Having foam-rolled my right leg as best I could—lower and upper leg; front, back and sides—I gave up for the day.

As I got to my feet, I recall being surprised that my foot felt 'different'. I couldn't quite put my finger on it, but it already felt a little freer and less restricted. It also didn't hurt as much.

I left the gym and went off for an easy evening stroll. Relatively speaking, it was like walking on air. The difference was already that apparent. It was still sore, but something positive was definitely 'afoot'!

My right leg was cramp free

That night I went to bed and, as always, the cramps hit, *but only in my left leg.* The enormity of that realization only dawned on me the following morning. I was my normal exhausted self, but everything was very different. I knew that my foot was healing.

And then it hit me, THERE HAD BEEN NO CRAMPING IN MY RIGHT LEG (remember, it was my right leg that I had worked on so intensely the previous day, during the foam rolling session).

You can only imagine my excitement. I would gladly have spent 24 hours a day on that foam roller.

And that was just the beginning.

The wonder of this new dimension

The foam roller, through its targeting of our fascia, has the capacity to help restore the original synergy between our anatomy, physiology, and neurophysiology. This, in my opinion, is how it catalyses the deep-healing response.

It focuses us, like almost nothing else can, on what's going on inside our bodies. Its effectiveness can be attributed to its mechanical interaction with our fascia, *together with the powerful and engaging meditation which it spontaneously catalyses.*

This is not to say that we in any way discount the value of physiotherapists, chiropractors, kinesiologists, psychologists, and the like. Outside of injury and illness, though, the foam roller provides us with a simple everyday means to rid ourselves of cramps and take charge of our own wellbeing.

Foam rolling meditation

You can't experience the pain of a spasm, scar, or adhesion, which the foam roller has discovered, without *memorising* what it'll feel like once it's been *'rolled away'*. Without realising it, you're meditating on your memory of what it felt like *before* it was hurt.

You're recalling what it felt like to live in an earlier version of yourself. In this way, you're pre-empting your own healing, *which the roller then enables.*

As your mastery of the process evolves, you're able to recall, memorise, and restore, ever earlier versions of your physical self. Eventually, with your physical self, restored, it's down to recalling, memorising, and restoring, your core memories of *emotional wellbeing*—from *even earlier* versions of yourself. This could even take you back to your childhood.

It's at this point that you'll experience the joys of emotional release, as you unplug from the memories of physical and emotional trauma and abuse, which were hard-wired into your psyche from your past. You'll find yourself living in the present, with the feelings of wellbeing you last experienced in your childhood.

Finally, you'll recall and memorise, how it once felt to live, *connected with your spirit.* Slowly but surely, you'll *roll* yourself into a liberated and self-transformed being.

Then, as you persist with your foam-rolling, your appetite for personal growth will continues to escalate. You'll find yourself shifting your habits until they're in sync with your now self-created blueprint. You'll at last believe in your own uniqueness and your astonishing capacity for making a difference out there. Finally, you'll be reconnected with your purpose and the meaningful problem-solving talents you were born with, but convinced into denying.

Nothing splendid has ever been achieved, except by those who dared believe that something inside of them was superior to circumstance.

Bruce Barton

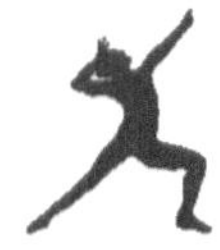

CHAPTER 6

Unexpected benefits

Wellbeing is the difference between living—and being truly, gloriously and authentically alive.

Goodbye restless leg syndrome

I've always suffered from restless leg syndrome. At night I simply could not keep my legs still. Terrible, if you happen to be in bed with a partner, especially when you already jackknife out of bed in the grips of leg cramps every five minutes!

My legs were still for the first time I could remember. Completely still.

No more distorted left foot

I put much of my initial healing effort with the foam roller, into my damaged right foot. It never crossed my mind, when I went to work on my left leg, that, apart from the cramps disappearing, my distorted left foot—the result of my motorbike accident in Lesotho all those years ago—would gradually heal too.

Miraculously, the unclogging and rebooting of the fascia, tendons and associated muscles, started releasing my foot. Within a month it was back to normal, after 30 years!

Cramp free, forever

Having finally healed my injured right foot (the pain has *completely* disappeared), it goes without saying that, except for when I haven't rolled for extended periods, I've lived cramp and pain free.

I'm running—fast—again, competing, nationally, in kayak marathons, and can drive as far as I like without being seized by cramps.

Don't forget your feet

An important point here is this; although most of the healing has undoubtedly taken place through the foam-rolling of my legs, I have not left my feet out. They continue to be an enormously important part of the healing puzzle.

Personally, I use a small wooden roller for the underside—and tops—of my feet. There are any number of these on the market. They work really well. You'll be surprised at how much residual pain and trauma lives on in your feet.

End of my knee pain

Lest I forget, I must mention that the knee pain I'd been suffering with because of a badly tracking kneecap, also disappeared. As soon as the iliotibial band was released through foam rolling (not by working on it directly—not a good idea—but by working on the tendons and muscles above and below it), my knee began tracking correctly and the pain dissolved.

Groin pain and headaches are no match for a foam roller

I've also suffered from a groin pain for the longest time. Groin injuries are notoriously hard to fix. Once I started foam rolling the insides of my thighs—right up to the knee joint—that pain also gradually dispersed.

Headaches, too, now seem to be a thing of the past. I started foam rolling my neck and back (very carefully!), and I now see that my toes really are connected to my head.

The compromised fascia in my legs, back and neck, together with damaged muscles and tendons, resulted in severe headaches. Damage to all these elements in the 'movement-chain' triggered adjustments and compensations all the way up to my head. Everything in our bodies is woven together in an intricate, interconnected and exquisite matrix.

Expanding the deep-healing process

Personally, I've tapped into nutrition, walking and running *barefoot,* and kayaking, as the value-adding elements to the foam-rolling process. There is truly nothing like grounding yourself, *daily,* by kayaking, and walking and/or running barefoot, preferably on grass or sand.

Apart from the feel-good factor, going barefoot helps restore our body's suspension-bridge-like *'superstructure'.* We engage tendons and muscles which we'd forgotten existed, and which help us regain our mobility, strength, flexibility, and wellbeing.

In summary

Wellbeing is the be-all and end-all of meaningful, joy-filled living. Without wellbeing it's difficult to find joy and meaning in anything.

Feelings of wellbeing are liberating. They inspire us to step into the flow of possibility, and to reach higher and further than we thought we could...

◆◆◆

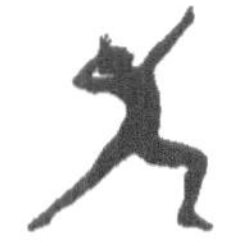

CHAPTER 7

New life

---

*Is there anyone so wise that they might
learn from the experience of others.*

The miracle of it all

With everything rebooted, I experienced the thrill and excitement of a little kid about to go off on holiday. I still lie in my bed and marvel at the miracle of it all. And it had all happened 'by accident'.

What if I'd never had a foot sore enough to want to do something about it? What if I'd never discovered the magic of foam rolling—beyond improving my athletic performance? And what if I'd discovered this all 20 years earlier? Life could have been so very different.

Incidentally, using the foam roller 20 years back was just too sore. I never even started, because my pain wasn't sufficiently debilitating at the time, to make me want to push through the initial discomfort of using the roller. And, of course, I'd never made the connection between my cramps and pushing through the pain barrier.

The benefits are simply endless

Do you find yourself wrapping a blanked around your legs and placing a hot-water bottle under your feet? It could be that you're constantly cold because you have compromised circulation in your legs and feet. Foam rolling could help you, under careful supervision *(especially if you have atherosclerosis or peripheral artery disease).*

Of course, you can never get around the fact that you'll need to optimize your diet and improve your exercise regime. You'll also need to keep foam rolling at least twice a week, and *move* for at least 5 minutes in every 30. This will help you sustain your cramp-free status.

Eventually, you'll regain 100%—or close to—mobility, strength, flexibility, speed and fitness. Plus, you'll experience many other priceless, *'unique to you',* health benefits.

Improvise until you have the right foam roller

You can even use a glass coke bottle—very carefully—as an interim roller (on a carpet, or yoga mat). A frozen oval-shaped water bottle works too, for a while.

Tennis balls can be useful for areas that are difficult to access with a foam roller (such as the neck and lower back). What some people do is to place two tennis balls in a sock, and tie it off. They then position the balls in the sock to apply pressure on either side of the spine, by lying on them, and gradually moving them from bottom to top.

Ideally though, you need a roller (various options are available for these hard-to-reach areas). From my experience, it's the repeated 'rolling' which does the trick.

Get creative!

Permanently catalysing the deep-healing response

Personally, I've discovered—again quite incidentally—that as my healing has accelerated, there have been many other unexpected spin-offs. I've alluded to it, but let me be clear on this; *I feel better on every possible level.*

Physically, I'm incredulous at the strides that I'm making daily. At 62, I can get up and run at any point in my day. I couldn't even dream of doing this before, without either damaging a muscle or hurting my knee. I love running barefoot on grass and sand now (previously, it was unthinkable).

My head is clear and (mostly) headache free, given that there are far fewer blockages in my neck and throughout my body.

Emotionally and spiritually, I feel consistently more upbeat, resilient, and connected. It's as if there really are no limits.

Accompanying these positive spin-offs, is the desire to consistently improve my nutrition—maximize my physical capabilities—so that I can continue to climb mountains, run freely, play, dance, and paddle rivers and oceans.

What's more, I'm more committed than ever to making a difference in other people's lives.

In combination then, it's about catalysing the deep-healing response through foam rolling, deep nutrition, light living, quality sleep, positive daily rituals (meditation, prayer and relaxation), and a varied exercise routine.

Add to the mix, engaging more actively with friends and family, and making a difference out there, and see the results for yourself.

Be sure to buy the right foam roller

Ideally, go out and buy a foam roller right away. They're inexpensive, and available at most sports and outdoor shops.

The beauty of the foam roller is that, once you have the basics, you can easily improvise your way forward.

The objective of this book is to help you make the connection between your muscle cramps, your aches and pains, your state of mind, and the need for foam-rolling. It's a profound 'life make-over'.

As a rule of thumb, do more rolling than you think you can, endure more pain than you think you can possibly bear—and roll from the less painful parts to those that are more painful. Gradually apply more pressure.

Then leave that area alone for a bit, while you use the roller elsewhere on your body. You'll be pleasantly surprised at how quickly your body will respond to your efforts, as painful as they may be, initially.

Be inspired

Like me, you can use your pain and circumstances as your inspiration to finally break free, and fly. Just like me, you may well have become who you've been socialized into believing you are; limited, stunted, and stuck with your unique mix of physical and emotional pain.

The good news is that you can undo the negative self-talk, and re-imagine your life. You can become who you've always known you can be.

It'll all make sense to you as you work your way through the process.

Stop thinking and talking about it, and there is nothing you will not be able to do.

Zen paradigm

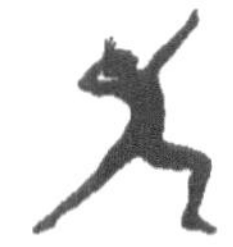

CHAPTER 8

Your life, your way

---

*We either live with the challenge of
discipline, or the misery of regret.*

It's your life

Now that you're the lead character in your life, it's time to be fully accountable and chart your own path.

To remind myself, daily, of who I am and the path I'm on, I've created *'My Destiny Oath'*. It's my lifetime contract with myself. I'm going to share it with you, in the hope that it'll inspire you to create something similar:

My Destiny Oath

I am the brightest star in my sky.

Every day I step into The Flow and shine with every fibre of my being.

Every day I live with the joy of who I have become, and the inspiration for who I am becoming.

I choose to live with love and meaning.

Occasionally I falter. That's ok.

For me, greatness is not a given, but I'm DARING GREATLY…

John Dickinson

CHAPTER 8

**The final inspiration is an extract from 'THE TAO OF POOH'
by Benjamin Hoff:**

*Let's find a Way Today
That can take us to tomorrow—
Follow that Way,
A Way like flowing water.*

*Let's leave behind
The things that do not matter,
And turn our Lives
To a more important chapter.*

*Let's take the time,
Let's try to find
What real life has to offer.
And maybe then
We'll find again
What we had long forgotten.
Like a friend,
True 'til the end,
It will help us onward.*

*The sun is high,
The road is wide
It starts where we are standing.
No one knows how far it goes,
For the road is never-ending.*

*It goes away,
Beyond what we have thought of.
It flows away,*

Away like flowing water.
"Perfect!" I said, "I knew you could do it".
"Have we reached the end?"
Asked Piglet.
"Yes", I replied, "I suppose so".
"It seems to be the end," said Pooh.
"It does, and yet—"
"Yes, Piglet?"
"For me, it also seems like a
Beginning."

Thank you so much for reading my book

Here's to your priceless health, and your future—cramp and pain free!

Wishing you well!

John Dickinson

♦♦♦

Endorsements

There are now many people who, having spoken to me, or read this book, are using this process with a new level of intensity and purpose. And they are celebrating the results.

Stuart Letton's experience is particularly close to me—because it was the very first. Stuart and his wife, Anne, who were travelling around the world on their yacht, arrived on our doorstep on 17 January 2022 on an overland adventure bike. They were using it to tour South Africa.

A week or so before this, they'd stopped at a traffic light and Stuart had put his foot out into thin air (there had been a drop-off that he hadn't anticipated). He'd done his best to save the bike going over, but to no avail; Stuart, Anne and bike tumbled to the ground. He hurt his back and hip in the process.

By the time they reached us, Stuart had tried everything to alleviate his suffering, but he was still in a lot of pain. When they left 48 hours later, after using my cramp-healing solution, his pain had largely been relieved; he was moving freely and sitting easily.

Although his wasn't specifically a cramp issue, my solution proved to be just as useful. I wasn't surprised; leveraging the rationale of the interconnectedness of all the different muscle groups, tendons and fascia in our bodies can help for a wide variety of injuries and conditions.

'It literally stares you in the face!' he said, 'I cannot believe that I never made the connection before.'

Sally Taylor's is a more recent success story. In her sixties, Sally suffered with the pain and frustration of nightly leg cramps—and occasional day cramps—for more years than she could remember. Within days of being introduced to my cramp healing solution, she was cramp free. Now, months later, she's still celebrating her newfound freedom.

Acknowledgements

Firstly, a huge thank you and a big hug to my partner, Tracey, whose support and inspiration has been inestimable. Thank you Trace!

Then, thank you to my long-suffering friend Michael, my harshest critic and greatest inspiration; my incredible friend Jill, who has always been there for me, and who introduced me to Jen, my editor; Jen, who brought the writing of this book to life – with her insights, persistence, passion and vision.

Disclaimer

Unless you have a serious underlying medical condition, it is unlikely that you'll experience any adverse side effects from this cramp-ridding, life-enhancing solution. Nevertheless, please exercise common sense and get a medical opinion if you believe that you may be at risk in any way.

For most of us, the biggest obstacle is not our medical condition. Rather, it's our conditioned mindsets which tell us that living cramp free is not an option. You'll need to let go of this misconception if you're serious about healing yourself, otherwise your limiting beliefs will deceive you into side-stepping a cramp-free future. You'll soldier on like you always have.

As always, there are no guarantees: your life, your choice.

This is not just about freeing yourself from the excruciating pain and frustration of your muscle cramps; it's about raising your game and living the rest of your life, differently.

Wishing you well!